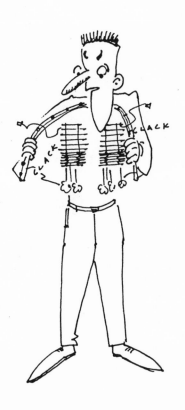

Hyperventilation Syndrome

Hyperventilation Syndrome
A Handbook
for Bad Breathers

DINAH BRADLEY

CELESTIAL ARTS

Berkeley • California

Cover design by Ken Scott
Text design by Lynn Meinhardt
Illustrations by Sally Hollis-McLeod
Typesetting by Ann Flanagan Typography

Originally published in New Zealand by Tandem Press, 1991

FIRST U.S. PRINTING 1992

Library of Congress Cataloging-in-Publication Data

Bradley, Dinah.
    Hyperventilation syndrome : a handbook for bad breathers /
Dinah Bradley.
        p.   cm.
    ISBN 0-89087-656-8
    1. Hyperventilation.   2. Hyperventilation—Psychosomatic
aspects.   3. Stress management.   I. Title.
RC776.H9B73   1992
616.2'08—dc20   91-37434
                                                        CIP

1   2   3   4   5   6   7   8   9   10   /   96   95   94   93   92

Contents

Foreword

In the Western world we are suffering from what has been called the paradox of health. Despite the fact that collective health has improved dramatically, perhaps because of technological advances and concentration upon preventative measures, there is a declining satisfaction with personal health. Many people report disturbing somatic symptoms and feelings of general illness.

One of the major reasons is the widespread commercialization of health, and the media's increasing focus on health issues, creating apprehension, insecurity, and alarm about disease, real or imagined.

A consequence of such tension is the condition of chronic hyperventilation, or Hyperventilation Syndrome. Although known about for many years, it has been largely ignored as a diagnostic alternative, resulting in extensive investigations that heighten the patient's anxiety. A bewildering collection of seemingly unrelated symptoms can be provoked by this condition, and recognition of its presence by health professionals is important, not only because reassurance can be given, but because treatment is simple and usually very effective.

In this monograph Dinah Bradley has beautifully presented the symptoms of Hyperventilation Syndrome and the therapy options available. Her book is very timely, as it seems more important now than ever to prevent extensive and expensive medical investigations and to get patients back to feelings of good health. Above all, it highlights the need for health professionals to have better communication with patients, to understand and help conquer their fears and anxieties.

This book will not only be appreciated by thousands of patients who will recognize themselves in its pages, it will also be very helpful to all those looking after the chronically ill. I wish it the success it deserves.

John Henley, MB, ChB, FRACP

Acknowledgments

Grateful thanks to Helen Benton and Bob Ross for their help, enthusiasm, and decision to be the first publishers of this book.

Heartfelt thanks, too, to Dr. John Henley for his help and encouragement, and to my physiotherapy colleagues.

I would like to acknowledge the research material by British physiotherapists A. Pilgrim and D. Innocenti, and the brilliant literature by chest physician L. C. Lum, MA, MB, FRCR, FRACP; and by P. G. F. Nixon, FRCP, whose clear and in-depth views were so valuable and inspiring.

Special thanks to Sally Hollis-McLeod for her superb cartoons.

Finally, I must mention the many patients who helped me experiment, formulate, and shape the BETTER breathing program, especially Rosa, who goaded me into producing this book.

Dinah Bradley

Introduction

The idea to write this book came about very shortly after I started a respiratory physiotherapy service for outpatients at the base cardiothoracic hospital in Auckland. Dealing mostly with asthma and other acute or chronic chest disorders, I was astonished by the high percentage of "bad breathers" with stress-related symptoms who appeared at the clinics.

Most of my previous twenty years as a physiotherapist had been spent with hospital inpatients—people in pajamas—who often had good reason to be breathing nervously; after major surgery, for instance, or because they were suffering from neurological or heart diseases, or from chest problems. Along with rehabilitation, a large part of my work involved breathing retraining and teaching stress management and relaxation methods to patients whose tension may have been delaying recovery or making existing symptoms worse.

I had no idea of the extent of disordered breathing—Hyperventilation Syndrome (HVS)—out in the wider world, away from hospitals. I should have, however, after researching and co-writing *Becoming Single—A Resource Book for the Newly Separated*. Most of the dozens of people I spoke to not only breathed chaotically while relating their marriage breakup stories, but many continued to hyperventilate habitually, long after the bad times were over.

It was a small, irate, elderly woman who made me finally decide to write this guide for hyperventilators. At the end of our first consultation, she clutched me by the collar and said: "Why hasn't anyone *explained* this to me before! I've learned more in the last hour than I discovered in thirty bloody years of going to the doctor... being fobbed off with pills... sent for tests for this and that... treated like a silly nuisance. *Give me something I can read about it!*"

After extensive searching for client-based information offering practical help, I drew a blank. Dozens of self-health books gave advice on breathing, but usually briefly, and at the end of the book, and in such a general way that people with disordered breathing would not have found it helpful (or worse, it would have exacerbated their symptoms).

Using research articles in various medical journals, along with my own twenty years of clinical experience, I devised a recovery program based on breathing retraining, tension release through talk and relaxation, enjoyable recreational exercise, and rebuilding confidence in the individual's ability to adapt to changes, loss, and stress.

Described by Claude Lum as "the great mimic," Hyperventilation Syndrome reproduces many baffling signs of all sorts of diseases. It may be hard to believe at first, let alone accept, that bad breathing can bring forth such devastating symptoms.

Both conventional and alternative medicine have let hyperventilators down. Written off with prescriptions for tranquilizers, antidepressants, and sleeping pills by busy GPs, many HVS sufferers come to rely on drugs to make sure they know exactly *how* they are going to feel each day and to blot out their typically erratic feelings of being well / not well / not bad, thanks / terrible.

As with all drugs, whether prescription or naturo-pathic, make sure *you* know *exactly* what you are putting down your throat. A good practitioner—orthodox or alternative—will be happy to give patients full informa-tion about the prescribed drug or natural remedy being offered. Ask to see the literature about the effects, side-effects and contra-indications. It's up to the patient to ask, and up to the doctor or health practitioner to answer to his or her satisfaction.

Hurt, confused, or annoyed by the orthodox "treat-ments" offered, some HVS sufferers resort to alternative therapies—aura cleansing, holistic pulsing, metaphysical healing, and iridology, to name a few—which are some-times accompanied by big bills, spartan diets, and expen-sive courses of vitamins. But the basic problem, Hyper-ventilation Syndrome, is not being diagnosed, or treated.

Breathing, like blinking, is an automatic activity that can also be controlled at will. One way to break the cycle of tension / over-breathing / anxiety / distress symptoms is to work on the one factor in the cycle that *can* be con-trolled by you: breathing.

Human beings are designed to react spontaneously to sudden dangers. We are less well adapted, though, to coping with prolonged stresses, and modern life is lit-tered with these. Fear of war, disease, isolation, or losing one's job are worries that rarely disappear after a good-night's sleep. In fact, nagging anxiety leads to broken sleep and transient feelings of unwellness, which results in further stress and altered breathing patterns.

After reading through this book—it is designed to be

read at a sitting—draw up a plan for yourself. Place in order the things that need attention, and discuss the plan with family and friends. Remember, there is no quick "cure." Allow time and patience to recover, to regain equilibrium and confidence, and to practice better breathing.

ONE
What is
Hyperventilation?

Hyper = too much, excessive, over the top.
Ventilation = the flow and movement of fresh air.

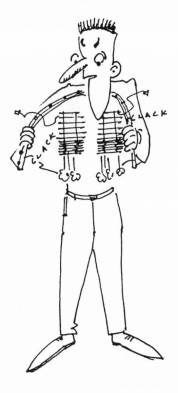

Hyperventilation means using the lungs to move more air in and out of the chest than the body can deal with.

Rapid or "over" breathing is a normal reaction in the short term to fever and acute infections, sudden exertion, fright, or intense emotion (such as love, rage, pain, or tears). But if it goes on for too long, unpleasant, bizarre, and sometimes even crippling symptoms can appear:

- Erratic heartbeats and / or chest pain.
- Breathless "attacks" at rest, for no apparent reason.
- Frequent sighing and / or yawning.
- Irritable coughing and chest tightness.
- Dizziness and "spaced out" feelings.
- "Pins and needles" or numbness in lips, fingertips, and toes.
- Gut disturbances—indigestion, nausea, wind, or irritable bowel.
- Muscle aches, pains, or tremors.
- Tiredness, weakness, disturbed sleep, and nightmares.
- Phobias.
- Clammy hands, flushed face, and feelings of high anxiety.
- Sexual problems.

These changes prime the body for action:

- Adrenalin pours into the bloodstream.
- Heart and breathing rates speed up.
- Muscles become tense.
- Eyesight and hearing sharpen.
- The pain threshold drops and pain is less intense.

This is how many people feel before a test or a job interview.

CASCADE OF SYMPTOMS

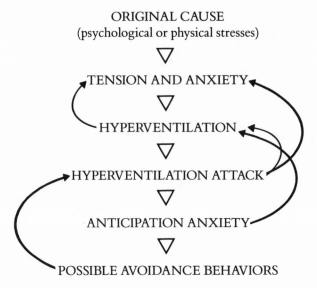

ORIGINAL CAUSE
(psychological or physical stresses)

▽

TENSION AND ANXIETY

▽

HYPERVENTILATION

▽

HYPERVENTILATION ATTACK

▽

ANTICIPATION ANXIETY

▽

POSSIBLE AVOIDANCE BEHAVIORS

Many people exploit controlled hyperventilation—before battle or competition (for example, the haka) or during religious festivals—to induce trance. New Age psychotherapy techniques such as rebirthing use it as a therapeutic tool. Uncontrolled or prolonged hyperventilation, however, can become dangerous.

How does this happen?

The exchange of air we breathe *in* (oxygen) and breathe *out* (carbon dioxide) is balanced by the lungs. Hyperventilation upsets this vital balance because more carbon

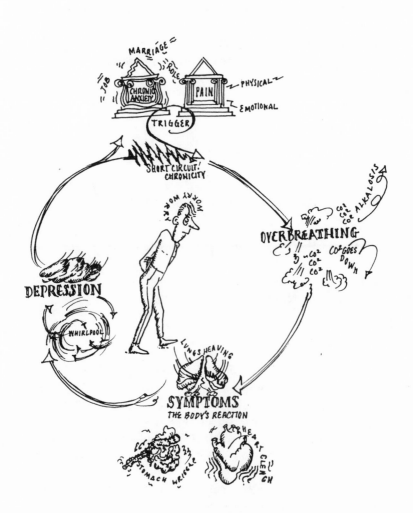

dioxide is breathed out than normal, and carbon dioxide levels in the blood start to drop. This upsets the normal acid / alkaline balance (pH) of the blood, and as a result the body becomes more alkaline than normal. This is known as respiratory alkalosis.

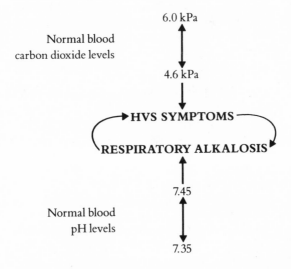

If carbon dioxide levels in the blood fall further with continued over-breathing, body cells begin to produce lactic acid to try and balance the pH of the blood and correct the alkalosis. The body's metabolism begins to suffer. Exhaustion and chronic tiredness soon follow, with feelings of depression—all typical signs of hyperventilation syndrome.

In a terrible Catch 22 cycle, natural anxiety about symptoms increases the tendency to over-breathe, further increasing respiratory alkalosis, which leads to more unpleasant or frightening symptoms.

Not only nerve cells are affected. Smooth muscle cells are galvanized into action by lowered carbon dioxide levels, which leads to tightening or constriction of the blood vessels. The heart and pulses start pounding, and the hyperventilator may feel panic-stricken with palpitations and chest pain. The brain may have its oxygen supply cut by as much as 50 percent, making it difficult to think, concentrate, or even feel part of this planet. Ultimately, all systems in the body are affected, leading to a puzzling constellation of symptoms.

Carbon dioxide, far from being just a "waste gas" at the end of the respiratory cycle, is actually a powerful governor of many of the body's functions. It is also the chief controller of the diameter of the blood vessels supplying the brain.

Why does this happen?

Everybody reacts in different ways to daily stresses and strains. For many people, life in the 1990s has been full of change and uncertainty. Adapting to change often brings with it anxiety, especially if the changes are unwanted (as in marriage breakdown, money worries, failure at school or on the job). Feelings of helplessness and loss of personal control over events, even over small things, can corrode self-esteem and confidence. Anxiety levels soar higher, and with them adrenalin levels, heart rate, and nervous tension—all fueled by overactive lungs.

Is hyperventilation a new syndrome?

Over the centuries many observations have been made about "the breath of life." Hippocrates, the "father of

Western medicine," in the fifth century B.C. noted: "The brain exercises the greatest power in mankind . . . but the air supplies sense to it."

Buddhism, which originated in the fifth century B.C. in India, had detailed accounts of breathing techniques to sustain health. These methods spread throughout Asia, and are best known in the twentieth century as yoga.

In ancient China, Taoism also had respiratory physiotherapy methods that combined breathing with relaxation and exercise to harmonize the various body systems, such as heart rate, circulation, digestion, and breathing. Movement and rest were evenly balanced. (The Chinese word for the interaction of exercise and rest literally translates as "feeding.")

Apart from well-observed accounts of swooning heroines and thunderstruck heroes in seventeenth- and eighteenth-century literature, little was understood about the link between over-breathing and ill-health in the West. Florence Nightingale, the "mother of nursing," was told she had heart disease when she suffered chest tightness, pain, and anxiety, and lived the latter half of her life as a semi-invalid. That she lived until she was ninety years old makes it unlikely that heart disease was her major problem.

The first detailed medical account of Hyperventilation Syndrome was published in 1871 by a doctor who had recorded his studies of 300 soldiers during the American Civil War. He pinpointed their "disabling shortness of breath and irritable heart" and the "oppression" of breathing, and thought that the source of the problem lay in the heart. By the First World War the condition was commonly known as "soldier's heart" syndrome. American doctors working with the British Medical Corps rejected this name, partly for psychological reasons, but mainly because signs of true heart disease were rarely found.

Some soldiers discovered a method of mimicking the syndrome's symptoms (not realizing that a few minutes' heavy breathing would have done the trick) by ingesting gunpowder, or "biting the bullet," in an attempt to escape from the horrors of war. This risky method was soon replaced by a much more permanent escape—death by firing squad—if soldiers were caught with gunpowder on their breaths.

Dr. T. Lewis, who coined the terms "soldier's heart" and "effort syndrome" in the 1920s, described the syndrome as "one of the commonest chronic afflictions of sedentary town dwellers."

Further research in the 1930s and 1940s increased knowledge about the physiology behind Hyperventilation Syndrome, but emphasis was still on it being secondary to primary neurotic or anxiety disorders ("the vapors"). Breathing into a paper bag (rebreathing exhaled carbon-dioxide-rich air) became a popular treatment for acute attacks of hyperventilation. No theater would be without a paper bag in the wings for stage-fright victims, frozen in respiratory alkalosis (terror) before making their entrance.

While still widely used for treating acute "panic attacks," the paper-bag technique is of no use to habitual hyperventilators because it fails to correct the basic cause —bad breathing. It also makes chronic hyperventilators dependent on something outside themselves—a crutch they might panic about being without—and who wants to be addicted to brown paper bags? In fact it can be extremely dangerous if people with acute asthma panic and try to control their rapid wheezy breathing in this way. At least one person is on record as breathing their last breath into a brown paper bag before expiring during a severe asthma attack.

Opinion is still divided today as to the true origins and definitions of Hyperventilation Syndrome. One camp treats the psyche first and lets the breathing take care of itself; the other emphasizes retraining of breathing rate and pattern (and rebalancing blood gases) and lets the psyche take care of itself.

This book attempts a combination of both approaches.

Further Reading

The Chinese Art of Healing, Stephen Palos (Bantam Books, New York, 1972).

From Medicine Man to Freud, Jan Ehrenwald (Dell Publishing, New York, 1956).

"Hyperventilation Syndrome: Infrequently Recognised Common Expressions of Anxiety and Stress," Gregory Margarian, *Medicine*, vol. 64, no. 4, 1982.

"Hyperventilation: The Tip of the Iceberg," Claud Lum, *Journal of Psychosomatic Research*, vol. 19, 1976.

"Hyperventilation and Cardiac Symptoms," P. G. F. Nixon, *Internal Medicine*, vol. 10, no. 12, 1989.

TWO
What Sort of People Develop HVS?

All sorts, and at all ages.

Children are not exempt. Behavioral problems may be the first indication, and checking children's chests often reveals effortless, rapid upper-chest breathing, fueling HVS symptoms.

Women in labor often hyperventilate for long periods during rapid, painful contractions. In these circumstances over-breathing amplifies pain, making it more intense. Childbirth classes concentrate on breathing control and relaxation techniques to combat this.

People with asthma (15 percent of New Zealand's population) are particularly prone to bad breathing habits and poor relaxation responses. Two or three decades ago physiotherapy was a top priority for newly diagnosed asthmatics, but with more recent emphasis on drug control of symptoms, not many now benefit from learning breathing control, rest positions, and relaxation to counteract the stresses and strains of asthma. The same applies to people with heart disease and hypertension. They may suffer chronic anxiety about their disorder, and poor breathing patterns increase their symptoms and heighten fears.

Older people having difficulties facing retirement and adjusting to aging and erratic health are prime candidates for HVS.

The condition is surprisingly common amongst teen-agers, where pressures to conform (from parents), to suc-ceed (from teachers), and to "be cool" (from friends) can be an unbearable burden.

High achievers seem to be sitting ducks for developing HVS if they set their sights too high and fail to reach unrealistic aims.

Unfortunately, HVS is all too common in those who feel powerless, for whatever reason, and who punish themselves for their perceived failures.

Sex, age, and occupation are no barrier to HVS, as the following cases demonstrate. (Read through them again after you have finished the whole text.)

T, a 25-year-old woman, had recently moved to a new town and started a new high-pressure job where she was expected to be glamorous as well as clever. After a par-ticularly bad few days when she felt she was not coping, she started to sleep poorly and felt increasingly anxious and irritable.

A former champion tennis player, T coached young players one evening a week, and found to her alarm her fitness levels had dropped drastically, with aching mus-cles and slowed reactions. Normally fit and energetic, she began to feel chronically tired and depressed. Her doctor prescribed sleeping pills to help break the insomnia / anxiety cycle, but by now her symptoms had escalated to shortness of breath for no apparent reason—often at rest— and occasional tingling of lips and fingertips. For this her doctor prescribed a Ventolin inhaler, which was of no help. She periodically felt hot and clammy and was con-vinced she had a low-grade viral infection.

Her relationship with her boyfriend was becoming strained. She had completely lost interest in sex, and suspected that he thought she was being a hypochondriac.

Some months later, after suffering a minor knee-strain at tennis which needed treatment, T's physiotherapist noticed her frequent sighing and yawning and poor breathing pattern, and suggested an appointment with a respiratory physiotherapist. Her doctor supported this plan.

These signs were noted: her respiratory rate was 22 breaths a minute (10 to 14 breaths a minute is normal range) with a pulse rate of 90 beats a minute (average adult pulse rate is 72). She sighed eight times in two minutes (average adult sigh rate is once every five to ten minutes).

While checking her breathing patterns, T had to loosen her tight-fitting belt before she could expand and breathe with her lower chest and diaphragm. She revealed that most of her clothes for work were tight-fitting. (Hyperventilation Syndrome in the 1970s was also called the "Designer Jeans Syndrome"—tight jeans restricted diaphragmatic breathing and shallow, upper-chest rapid breathing became a habit.)

It took T several months to restore her breathing to a normal rate and pattern, with good days gradually starting to outnumber bad days as she put stress-management techniques into action at work (along with elasticized waistbands).

H, a 43-year-old secondary schoolteacher at a posh boys' school had had well-controlled mild asthma since childhood, but after a period of extra work at school he began experiencing anxiety attacks and bouts of shortness of breath for no particular reason. Thinking it was deteriorating asthma, he became depressed at his lack of physical fitness and coping abilities, and increased his asthma drugs.

When he was checked out by a chest physician, a hyperventilation component to his asthma symptoms was clearly seen. Even though H had previously been taught to breathe well, he was amazed when the physiotherapist pointed out his upper-chest/mouth-breathing pattern.

Before a prone-lying relaxation session his pulse rate was 96, his breathing rate was 22 per minute, and his peak flow measurement (the amount of air breathed out through a small device people with asthma use to measure wheeziness) was 480. After the session, his breathing rate was 12, his pulse 80, and his peak flow had improved to 620.

Over-breathing was making his asthma symptoms worse, and the discovery of his ability to help control tension and breathe correctly was enough to motivate H to change his faulty breathing pattern, practice regular relaxation, and improve his physical reserves with a graduated walking program.

O, a 54-year-old businessman, had suffered a very mild stroke from which he had completely recovered, but he was so anxious it would happen again, that he became extremely tense and depressed. Rapid breathing added real symptoms to his imagined ones.

O became very isolated and felt he was letting his family down. His wife had to drive him to his first appointment with the physiotherapist. He was restless, sighed three or four times a minute, and had cold, clammy hands. His breathing rate was 20 per minute in an upper-chest/ mouth-breathing pattern; his pulse was 84.

He immediately grasped the concept of over-breathing affecting blood-gas levels and causing such widespread symptoms, and after only two sessions was breathing well, driving again, and relieved of most of his crippling anxieties.

A, 13 years old, terrified the staff at her school as well as her parents with episodes of racing heart-rates, very rapid breathing (30 to 40 per minute), and fainting. After a number of trips by ambulance to Casualty, a respiratory physician diagnosed Hyperventilation Syndrome and mild asthma, and referred her to a respiratory physiotherapist for breathing retraining, stress management, and asthma education. It turned out that A was having problems adapting to her early blossoming into physical maturity well ahead of her classmates.

As is more common with teenage hyperventilators, fainting was the most dramatic symptom of A's habitual over-breathing. This stopped almost immediately once she got over the fear of the "attacks," understood the rationale behind them, and began using rest positions and controlled breathing to cope with sudden breathlessness. She continued to have outbreaks—before exams or during times of conflict—but had the skills to deal with the unpleasant symptoms at her command, *if she chose to.*

P was a tall, glamorous, 43-year-old woman who, two years ago, had given up a satisfying part-time job because of "poor health." She had suffered panic attacks while driving her car, and for about a year was unable to drive down one particular stretch of road.

She was now a full-time housewife and mother, and did absolutely everything for her husband and three teenage sons. She had recently painted the whole exterior of the family house by herself, but brushed that off as "nothing." Her sense of self-worth was at ground level, and her family had adapted to her diminished estimation of herself as their slave. P was chronically tired and had completely lost the ability to tell the difference between normal tiredness and exhaustion. She only took to her bed if she had "something wrong," which became increasingly common.

P's breathing rate at the first physiotherapy session was 25 per minute and her pulse rate was 90. She had attended ante-natal classes for the births of her children, remembered diaphragmatic breathing and found it easy to do, but very hard to sustain. Relaxation was also extremely difficult and it was decided to leave exercise off her program until diaphragmatic breathing was well established as a normal pattern and she had developed a good relaxation response.

A few days after the first session she telephoned to report that she felt worse than ever, and that trying to relax was a problem. At the next session it was decided to adopt a "listening-relaxing" approach. P loved music but had rarely listened to any in the past few years. She recorded the six Bach cello suites, each about twenty minutes long, on separate tapes and found listening to these while remaining still and totally relaxed a successful way to "let go." The music helped blot out the guilt she had previously felt when taking time out for herself to relax.

Low, slow breathing, rest, and relaxation were top priorities for the first month. Her family was very helpful, with the youngest son taking on the role of jester and keeping his mother supplied with jokes. P started a graduated walking program in the fifth week, and after eight sessions at the clinic she felt she had the skills needed to continue on her own. A few months later she rang to say that she had driven down the stretch of road that had terrified her—a personal goal achieved.

THREE
What is
"Good Breathing"?

Three groups of muscles are used for breathing:

The diaphragm
Tailor-made for each person to supply the right amount of air to the lungs during rest and normal activity, this strong, thin, flat sheet of muscle attached to the lower borders of the ribs, separates the chest from the gut. Shaped rather like an open umbrella, it flattens like a parasol to expand the lungs and draw in a sufficient air supply with very little effort.

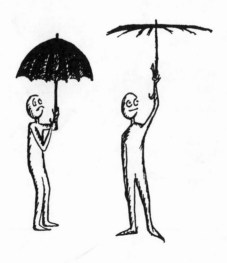

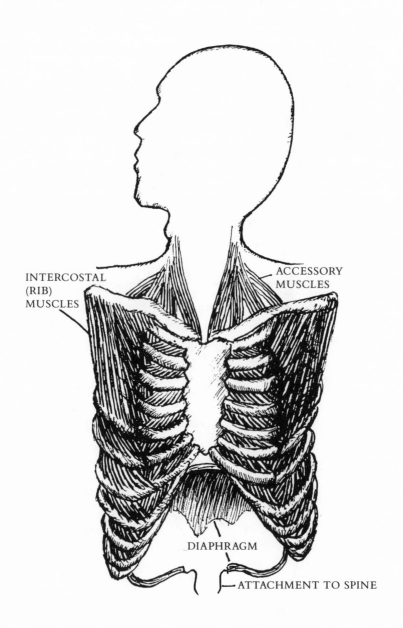

INTERCOSTAL
(RIB)
MUSCLES

ACCESSORY
MUSCLES

DIAPHRAGM

ATTACHMENT TO SPINE

The diaphragm also acts as a vital pump, helping the heart circulate blood up and down the body. Movement can vary from 1 centimeter at rest to 10 centimeters during vigorous activity. Diaphragmatic breathing is the most energy-efficient and relaxing way to breathe.

Chest or intercostal muscles
These attach between each rib and tighten to lift the ribs, like birds' wings, expanding the chest wall to draw in air and contracting to push it out. They are used more during moderate to strong effort and use about 20 percent more energy than the diaphragm.

Accessory muscles
These include shoulder and neck muscles used to tense the shoulders and lift the upper chest to help draw in extra air. They can be seen working after strenuous exercise or effort. (In hyperventilators, they can be seen working in breathing rates of 20-plus per minute.)

In normal, easy breathing, 70 to 80 percent of the work of respiration is done by the diaphragm. The lower chest or intercostal muscles do about 20 to 30 percent of the work. The accessory muscles are used during, and shortly after extremes of effort or stress. Habitual hyperventilators tend to reverse this ratio.

Oxygen and carbon dioxide levels, or blood gases, are kept in healthy balance by 12 regular breaths a minute (10 to 14 is an acceptable range)—two to three seconds to breathe in; three to four seconds to breathe out—moving about 600 cubic centimeters of air with each breath.

2 sec IW + 3 sec out = 5 secs
3 sec IW   4 sec out = 7 secs

Math!

10/min = 6 secs per cycle

$\frac{60}{10}$ = 6 secs / breath cycle (In - Out)

14/min = 4.3 secs / cycle

✗ 8.6 cycles

$\frac{60}{14}$ ≈ 4.29 ≈ 4.3

$\frac{60}{5 sec}$ = 12 cycles / min

21

Good breathing occurs when the respiratory rate is in this range, and when the diaphragm does the majority of the work, with little or no upper-chest movement at all.

GOOD BREATHER   BAD BREATHER

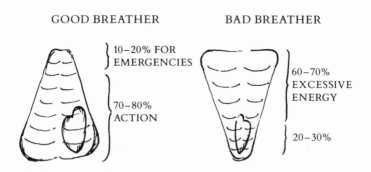

Nose-breathing is a major part of respiratory health. Air breathed in through the nose is:

- Warmed (lungs dislike cold, dry air).
- Moisturized (75 percent humidification of inhaled air occurs in the nose and throat, compared with 25 percent via the mouth).
- Filtered (inhaled dust and debris are caught by tiny nasal hairs not present in the mouth).

It is hard to hyperventilate for long while nose-breathing.

The combination of cold, dry, unfiltered air being drawn in larger-than-normal quantities into the upper chest causes several problems in the respiratory system:

GOOD   BAD

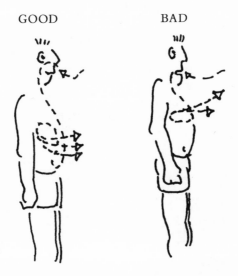

- Poor mixing and circulation of air throughout the lungs.
- Less efficient absorption and exchange of blood gases in the alveoli (air sacs).
- The body starts to suffer.

For people with persistent nasal problems who find it uncomfortable or too difficult to nose-breathe, and where nose drops, sprays, and medications have not helped, other treatment alternatives include:

- Physiotherapy. This offers non-invasive, painless, non-drug alternatives with shortwave or ultrasound electrical treatments.
- Acupuncture. One study reported a 70 percent success rate using this method to treat chronic rhinitis. The

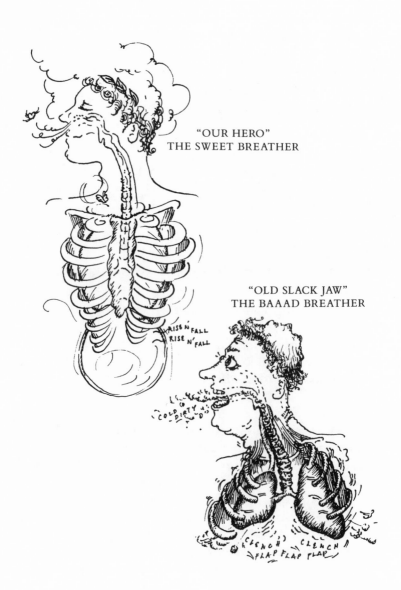

improvements lasted six or seven months, on average. If all else has failed, it *is* worth a try.

- Nasal washes. Stir a teaspoon of bicarbonate of soda and a teaspoon of salt into a glass of hot water. When cool, pour into a clean, empty nasal-spray bottle. Use as a "wash" two or three times a day.

Why do people become hyperventilators?

The respiratory center in the hind-brain responds to messages from different parts of the body as well as from the higher brain. After a bout of rapid breathing—whether from hard exercise, high emotions, or danger—the respiratory system gradually allows the breathing rate to slow down as the body regains balanced blood gases. However, for some under prolonged stress, the respiratory center slowly adapts to accept low or fluctuating carbon dioxide levels and respiratory alkalosis. So, while various parts of the mind and body may feel extremely unhappy about the blood-gas imbalance, the respiratory center rides roughshod over any distress signals it receives, and keeps on instructing the lungs to breathe hard and fast.

The causes of this condition can be mechanical, occurring after lung surgery or in lung diseases that cause air-flow disturbances (e.g., tuberculosis or bronchiectasis).

The problems can start after illnesses like viral chest infections, pneumonia, glandular fever, and ME (myalgic encephalitis), or post-viral fatigue syndrome.

HVS can appear during or after emotional upheavals:

- Death of a partner / lover / family member.
- Separation and divorce.
- Losing a job or being fired.
- Changes of status / growing up / aging.
- Moving to a different town.
- Living in a war zone.

Exercise, too, can trigger hyperventilation attacks where high stress levels and low physical reserves combine to bring on a sense of panic.

What does it feel like to hyperventilate?
The most common phrases used by hyperventilators are:

- "I thought I was going to pass out—I couldn't seem to take the next breath *in*."
- "I never seem to be able to take a satisfying breath."
- "I've never felt quite the same since my operation / accident / breakup . . ."
- "I really thought I was going crazy . . ."
- "I thought I was *dying* . . ."

In sudden attacks, people usually are aware of their heaving upper-chest breathing and high anxiety, but are quite unable to slow down. The strange symptoms that might follow, such as dizziness, tingling fingers and lips, and loss of concentration, lead some to dire conclusions. (See Woody Allen going for a brain scan in the film *Hannah and Her Sisters*.)

Those who go to their doctor are usually prescribed a tranquilizer after a checkup and given reassurance that "nothing is wrong." For some, this may be enough to break the cycle. But others who find their strange symptoms still lurking may start to imagine:

HEART ATTACK!
BRAIN TUMOR!
BOWEL CANCER!

Do they go back to their doctor? Do they write their wills?

Once the breathing pattern becomes centered in the upper chest and away from the diaphragm, more widespread and frightening symptoms begin to be felt.

The hazards of heavy breathing

- Habitual mouth-breathers develop irritable upper airways, with the risk of repeated throat infections. A very common sign of hyperventilation is repeated throat-clearing—the *A-Hrrmm* bug.
- Chronic hyperventilation triggers increased histamine levels in the blood. Sweaty palms and armpits, clammy skin, and a flushed face are all signs of this. People with allergies such as hayfever, skin rashes, food intolerances, or asthma find their symptoms are much worse.
- Response to pain is amplified too: stiffness and tension in muscles, tendons, and joints, brought about by bad breathing, starts to feel like full-blown rheumatism.
- Heart disease-type symptoms, like chest tightness or pain or pounding pulses, can be downright terrifying.
- Mental fuzziness, headaches, or loss of concentration can erode self-confidence, especially if work suffers.

- Making love can become a nightmare—for both partners—if the "heavy breathing" needed to have an orgasm leads to a panic attack.
- Vivid dreams, nightmares, and disturbed sleep patterns commonly accompany hyperventilation, making for round-the-clock distress.

The cycle is completed. Almost every system in the body suffers. Anxiety and fear of frightening symptoms drives the respiratory center into top gear.

Hyperventilation Syndrome gives full throttle to the fear... and the symptoms... and bewilderment.

Further Reading

"Acupuncture Therapy in Allergic Rhinitis," P. Chari, *American Journal of Acupuncture*, vol. 16, no. 2, 1988.

"Behavioural Breathlessness," J. B. L. Howell, *Thorax*, 45, 1990.

"Chronic Hyperventilation Syndrome," D. H. Innocenti, in *Cash's Textbook of Chest, Heart and Vascular Disorders*, ed. P. A. Downie (4th edition, Faber and Faber, London, 1987).

"Dyspnoea: A Sensory Experience," R. Schwarztzstein *et al., Lung*, vol. 168, 1990.

Respiratory Physiology, John B. West (4th edition, Williams and Wilkins, Baltimore, 1990).

FOUR
Is HVS
Very Common?

Relatively little research has been published on Hyperventilation Syndrome, but British chest physician Claude Lum, who has done the most extensive clinical work on the subject over the last twenty-five years or so, has found that the problem is extremely widespread. About 12 percent of any normal population are bad breathers, and Lum maintains that the numbers are increasing.

GPs generally agree that they find 10 to 12 percent of their patients display signs of chronic hyperventilation. Specialists attract higher numbers, estimating that 50 to 70 percent are habitual over-breathers. No figures are available from alternative healthcare sources.

Various studies from emergency, coronary care-unit admissions for chest pain have revealed that 30 to 40 percent of the suspected heart-attack victims had absolutely nothing wrong with their hearts.

How does a doctor know if symptoms are caused by HVS?
After a thorough checkup—which, depending on symptoms, could involve anything from a brain scan to a barium enema—nothing sinister has been uncovered, the doctor may test for HVS by:

- The 12-Breath Test. The patient is asked to stand and take 12 rapid breaths, which many sufferers are amazed to find reproduces exactly their distressing symptoms.
- The Think Test. Breathing patterns are watched as the patient talks about symptoms and anxieties. Most people can pinpoint an event that caused them extreme stress, which when they bring it to mind, along with their increased rate of breathing, also brings on most of their symptoms.

Other, more hi-tech methods of diagnosis are available, but because blood-gas levels fluctuate in chronic hyperventilators, it may be difficult to pick up the problem from a single test. Often patients have already been through batteries of stressful or painful tests, and many doctors prefer the direct 12-Breath or Think Tests rather than subject them to more complex tests.

Unfortunately for those whose HVS symptoms include chest pain, it is one of the hardest to reproduce in the safety of the doctor's presence by over-breathing "on command."

There are three main types of chest pain associated with HVS:

- Sharp pains felt while breathing in from pressure on the diaphragm from a bloated stomach, caused by "air gulping," which results in spasms of the diaphragm and pain.
- Dull aching pain with chest-wall soreness, most often felt after exercise. This is due to overuse of chest wall (intercostal) and accessory muscles, which tire easily and hurt.

- Heavy pain behind the breast bone radiating to the neck and arms. This happens when the blood supply to the heart muscle itself is reduced by HVS stress / anxiety and spasms of the coronary arteries.

In all three types of pain, many stresses (physical, social, and emotional) may combine with hyperventilation to bring on chest pain—stresses not found in the security of the doctor's rooms.

What can be done for hyperventilators?

Unfortunately, many doctors, once they find nothing clinically wrong, fail to take account of the disabling effects of HVS or its bad-breathing origins. Being told "Go away. There's absolutely nothing wrong," may be briefly reassuring, but only until symptoms materialize again. (See Woody Allen *after* the results of his brain scan in *Hannah and Her Sisters*.)

Often symptoms seem infinitely worse. If no one believes the symptoms are real, does it mean that it's all in the mind? Or worse still, incurable. People who already have disorders such as asthma, heart disease, or chronic pain that may be made worse by bad breathing are frequently loaded with extra drugs for the existing condition instead of being treated for the coexisting hyperventilation problem.

This is assuming that your doctor is even aware of HVS. Hi-tech medical training in recent years offers only passing mention of the subject to trainee doctors. This results in doctors focusing only on symptoms, and in early pigeonholing of their patients as suffering from "anxiety neuroses," "depression," "hypochondriasis," or being "panic attack-prone." They then treat the *symptoms* of HVS, not the underlying over-breathing disorder (rather like prescribing skin lotion to someone with yellow jaundice).

The most commonly prescribed drugs for these symptoms are tranquilizers and anti-depressants, which act by burying the cause and leave the over-breathing component untreated. This exposes the patient to the added risks of addiction, and further loss of self-confidence.

Well-informed doctors refer their patients with persistent HVS to respiratory physiotherapists for assessment, treatment, and management of their breathing disorder. Long-term bad breathers may need many sessions in breathing retraining and sorting out the often complex side effects that have radiated from HVS and its legacy of symptoms. For instance, some chronic hyperventilators develop avoidance behaviors in an attempt to control their symptoms. Chronic anxiety can lead to phobias—most commonly, fear of open spaces (agoraphobia) or enclosed spaces (claustrophobia). Common, too, is fear of travel; driving a car or fear of flying, for example. Anxiety about sex can lead to loss of desire through fear of failure or fear of not being able to cope with intense emotions. Referral for specialized treatment or counseling would be indicated if these problems remained deep-rooted.

Where to start?

One doctor has described HVS as "a diagnosis begging for recognition." Once correctly diagnosed, the treatment is simple and involves no needles, no drugs, and no pain. The six-step program in the second part of this book uses the acronym BETTER to cover important aspects of recovery:

- Breathing retraining
- Esteem
- Total body relaxation
- Talk
- Exercise
- Rest and sleep

The following six chapters outline one successful way to combat HVS and restore normal breathing patterns (and blood gases), and examine ways to help cope with the pressures that cause the problems.

Further Reading

"Demonstration and Treatment of Hyperventilation Causing Asthma," G. Hibbert and D. Pilsbury, *British Journal of Psychiatry*, vol. 153, 1988.

"Hypertension and Hyperventilation—a common combination that is rarely diagnosed," Norman M. Kaplan, *Cardiology Guide*, October 1989.

"Psychogenic Breathlessness and Hyperventilation," Claude Lum, *Update*, May 1987.

FIVE
Breathing Retraining

Nobody needs to be shown *how* to breathe, but many people are bad breathers, using their upper-chest muscles instead of their diaphragms.

For people with HVS, restoring a normal breathing pattern may take time and a lot of regular practice. Some are able to switch easily to low, slow, diaphragm breathing, while others may take months, sometimes up to a year, to change their ways. The following simple techniques will help turn you into a good breather, but if you continue to have problems you may need extra help from a respiratory physiotherapist.

The four basic steps to follow are:

- Becoming aware of faulty breathing patterns.
- Learning to nose-diaphragm breathe.
- Suppressing upper-chest movement during normal breathing.
- Reducing breathing to a slow, even, rhythmic rate (the average breathing rate for adults is about 12 breaths per minute; two to three seconds to inhale, three to four seconds to exhale).

Big versus deep breaths
People learn from a very early age, often at school, to stick out their chests and hold in their stomachs like soldiers

or beauty queens when asked to breathe. Ask anyone to take a *deep* breath and chances are that they will puff up their upper chest and take a *big* breath instead.

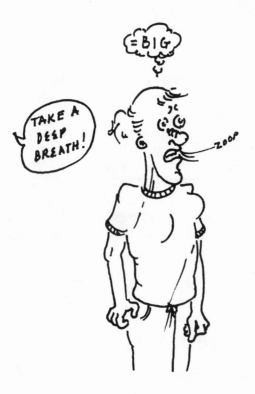

Try it. First, place the hand you write with on your stomach between your lower ribs and navel. Put the other hand on your breastbone, just below your collarbones (the Lung Ho salute, with apologies to Rewi Alley).

✿ THE LUNG-HO ✿
SALUTE

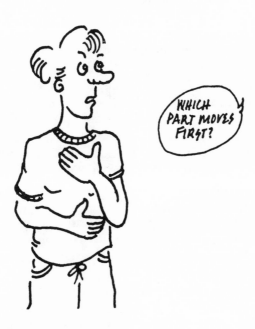

Take a *deep* breath and notice:

- Which part of your chest moved first?
- Which part of your chest moved most?
- Did you breathe in through your mouth or nose?

If you breathed in through your nose, your stomach expanded first and you felt almost no upper-chest movement, you are a good breather.

If you breathed in fast through your mouth, your upper chest heaved first and you felt little or no movement under your writing hand, or your stomach drew *in*, then you are a bad breather.

Strategies for breathing retraining

Practice lying comfortably on your back, head well supported with pillows or cushions. Let as much air as possible sigh out of your lungs *without pushing*. Shoulder and upper-chest relaxation is vital here.

With lips together, jaw relaxed, draw air slowly in through your nose, relaxing and expanding your waist so your stomach puffs up. Let the air "fall" out of your chest as the elastic recoil of your lower chest and diaphragm breathes air out *effortlessly*.

Take very small abdominal breaths at first, making sure you start each in breath with the diaphragm.

Mentally repeat to yourself: "Lips together, jaw relaxed, breathing low and slow."

Imagine a fine piece of elastic round your waist, stretching as you inhale; or think of breathing into your belt or waistband. Check chest movement using the Lung Ho salute.

If you find it hard to keep breathing low and slow, placing a heavy book on your stomach helps focus effort.

Timing

Once you feel confident about the breathing pattern, concentrate on the rate. Get the feel of how long two to three seconds are by counting silently (adding the word

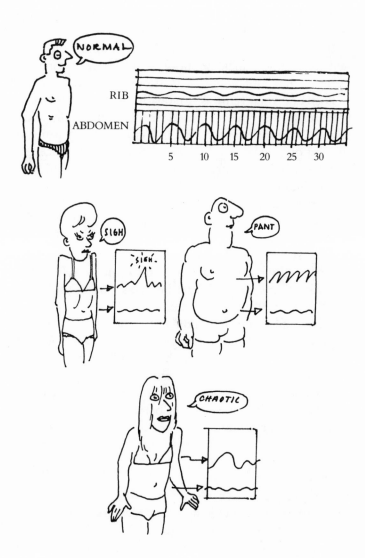

"hundred" after each number equates roughly to one second—one hundred, two hundred, etc.).

If you have been a very rapid breather for a long time, you may only manage a one-second *in*, two-second *out* cycle for the first few practice sessions.

Focus on the evenness, gradually increasing the time taken to breathe in and out. Breathing out usually takes slightly longer than breathing in, with a relaxed pause at the end of exhalation. This may be more pronounced in people with chest disorders such as asthma or chronic airway limitation (CAL).

Practice the new low, slow, breathing pattern lying on your side, sitting and standing. Try breathing this way while walking.

At first, if you have been addicted to mouth/upper-chest breathing, nose-diaphragm breathing will feel very peculiar. Some people describe it as "back to front" breathing.

It can take a long time and constant practice to get your diaphragm strong and working confidently. Don't be hard on yourself if you revert to bad breathing habits. Just concentrate on the next breath and getting it right.

Use the rest positions illustrated opposite when and wherever you become short of breath and need to focus on low, slow breathing.

How often?

Before you get out of bed every morning, lie on your back for a few minutes practicing relaxed low, slow breathing, to establish the pattern for the day.

During the day, check your breathing pattern with the Lung Ho salute, *every hour on the hour.* Constant repetition

REST POSITIONS

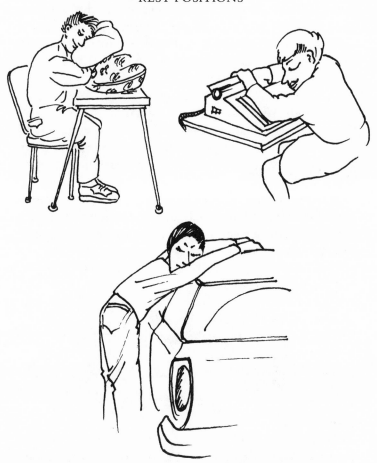

is the best way to reinforce your healthy breathing pattern.

In bed at night, repeat the morning breathing routine lying on your side to help you get to sleep.

As you become accustomed to breathing this way, the need to Lung Ho will be less. During stressful times though, it pays to check your breathing pattern and rate, and pay more attention to control.

Common mistakes and problems

Your diaphragm may be a bit jumpy at first, especially if it has been out of action for a long time. The muscle itself may need strengthening. If you find yourself breathing in a jerky, "staircase" fashion, mildly resisted breathing with a five-pound bag of rice or sugar (one woman found her iron made a perfect weight) on your upper stomach helps reinforce the good pattern. Try this lying on your back for ten minutes twice a day for a week.

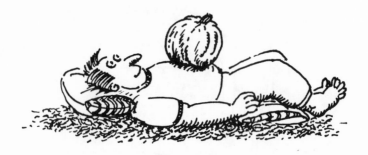

People on courses of steroid tablets, for whatever reason, need to pay special attention to keeping their diaphragm strong, as deconditioning, which happens in big muscle groups as well as the diaphragm, has been shown to occur during treatment. Strengthening exercises help restore muscle power.

Those with asthma—children and adults—also need to pay special attention to their breathing after a bout of wheezing. Breathing may be chaotic during an attack, switching from upper-chest to diaphragmatic, with little chance of good control; an increased respiratory drive is natural at this time. But using rest positions and reducing shoulder- and upper-chest muscle fatigue as much as possible helps combat the fear and anxiety that accompany asthma. Once the attack is over, reestablishing a low, slow, breathing pattern and suppressing upper-chest use must be top priority.

Your body will try to play all sorts of tricks to start over-breathing again. The urge to sigh, yawn, or "air-gulp," and race back to hyperventilation will seem overwhelming at times, and very uncomfortable at first. To help stop this from happening, try swallowing or holding your breath for two or three seconds anywhere in the breathing cycle and concentrate on the low, slow pattern.

Remind yourself that your respiratory center is frantically trying to make you hyperventilate again. But with regular and determined practice your respiratory center will readjust to restore normal blood pH levels and normal ventilation.

Another common trick is to "brace," or fill up the upper chest, holding in huge volumes of air while using the diaphragm to breathe in more. Breathing this way will make symptoms worse.

It is as important to suppress high, upper-chest breathing and relax shoulders and chest as it is to center breathing low and slow.

An excellent image to use in focusing on low, slow breathing is to imagine breathing through your heels.

When you feel your breathing going high (with sighs) remember to:

- Relax your shoulders by using a rest position.
- Keep lips together, jaw relaxed, shoulders down.
- Concentrate totally on low, slow breathing until you start to feel in, not out of, control.

It's over to you.

Further Reading

The Body in Question, Jonathan Miller (Jonathan Cape, London, 1978).

"CO_2 Response and Pattern of Breathing in Patients with Symptomatic Hyperventilation, Compared to Asthmatic and Normal Subjects," J. Hormbrey *et al.*, *European Respiratory Journal*, 1, 1988.

"Handling the Chronic Hyperventilation Patient," A. Pilgrim, *Physiotherapy*, vol. 72, no. 6, 1986.

Mechanisms of Body Functions, D. M. Easton (Prentice Hall, New Jersey, 1974).

SIX
Esteem

Most habitual hyperventilators suffer from a battered self-image, one of the first major casualties in an outbreak of HVS. Good days may be few and far between, and these are overshadowed by fear and loathing of bad days. Gradual erosion of confidence—feeling that you are letting people down—also adds to a general sense of lack of self-worth. Strong positive emotions like love, happiness, and laughter gradually get pushed aside by anger (often repressed), anxiety, and depression.

Most people get a lot of attention during times of major upheaval, such as after a birth, death, marriage, or separation. However, the cumulative effects of minor, everyday niggles are very often left unresolved and can build to major proportions if they are allowed. Learning to say "sorry, but no" to demands you know will overload you is a very important skill to master.

Loosening up, relaxing, and finding some humor in your life will prove that laughter—as well as being the best medicine—is also a powerful and non-toxic remedy. Laughter benefits the whole person, body and soul. A good laugh liberates petrified minds from repetitive, often negative, thought patterns. The body's immune system is boosted too. One humor researcher found increased levels of immunoglobulins (antibodies) were produced in people watching funny films, versus those watching dull documentaries. Laughter also seems to reduce output of the stress hormone adrenalin; and just as exercise releases opiopeptides (hormones that make you feel good), so does laughter. The final bonus is the immediate and exquisite relaxation that follows laughter.

Breaking the tension → HVS → anxiety → HVS cycle needs a firm commitment to changing your outlook as well as your breathing patterns. Language and choice of words play an important part here. To start, cross the word "should" out of your vocabulary.

Awareness of thought and speech patterns—with fragmented, illogical, and mostly negative phrases dominating—can be changed. If you catch yourself thinking things like, "I'll never be able to manage," or, "I'm always letting people down," gently question yourself—never? always?—and *think* about it. Break the line of despair.

Fear of losing control is especially strong in chronic hyperventilators. This often leads to repression of normal emotions, and the withholding of love, warmth, anger, or sadness. Unexpressed grief, fear, or resentment puts people in the fast lane to depression and withdrawal from everyday life.

At the risk of giving depression a good name, it *is* a fairly normal reaction to prolonged bouts of hyperventilation and resulting nasty symptoms. If there is nothing concrete to "cut out" or take a pill for, anxiety and depression are reasonable enough reactions to feeling constantly off-center. Being diagnosed as suffering from anxiety and depression is undermining enough. Unfortunately, treating the symptoms of these without first sorting out the basic breathing disorder is going to be of limited value to the individual, and of great expense to our health-care system. Chemical happiness in the form of prescribed tranquilizers and antidepressants must be approached with caution.

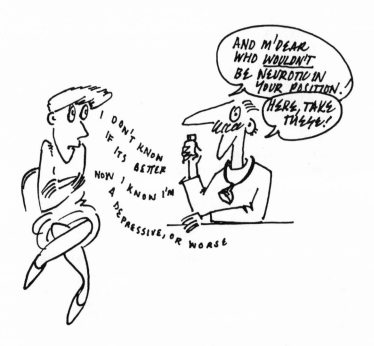

More sinister than the accompanying wearing away of self-esteem is the likelihood of turning hyperventilators into chronic invalids. After being shunted from specialist to specialist trying to find a diagnosis, and undergoing all sorts of sometimes risky investigations or drug therapies with no relief, is it surprising that anxiety and depression should become permanent members of the band?

Failure to recognize over-breathing, exhaustion, denial of normal tiredness, and abuse of stimulants like coffee and cigarettes (and worse) to boost flagging energy levels, is asking for trouble once your body starts signaling distress. Many people—mature, intelligent, clever people—are positively backwards at recognizing signs of exhaustion. These can include:

- Increased heart and breathing rate.
- Mental and physical restlessness and difficulty relaxing.
- Slowed reactions and reflexes.
- Inability to concentrate.
- Irritability and a tendency to fly off the handle.
- Loss of energy and stamina.
- Poor resistance to colds and flu.
- Loss of interest in sex.

Someone with a healthy self-image is much more likely to take notice of their body's reactions to tiredness, stress, and the early signs of exhaustion. Developing a sense of balance between effort (good for the ego), relaxation (physical and mental rejuvenation), sleep (recovery), and exercise (increasing physical reserves) is a good way to rebuild esteem for yourself and for others.

Good posture, too, is a very important ingredient in strengthening self-confidence. Try this regularly: imagine being suspended by a fine thread from the back of the top of your head; stretch up tall to prevent the phantom thread from breaking.

Always sit with your bottom snug against the back of the chair. Maintaining a lumbar hollow when sitting stops your upper spine from sagging and compressing your chest.

Apart from the mechanical advantages to the process of breathing itself, holding and carrying yourself well—standing or sitting—makes you feel in charge and physically confident.

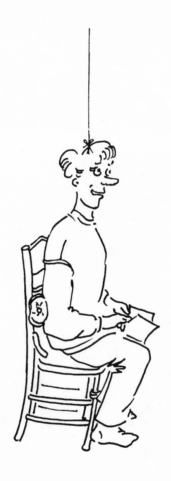

Another potent way of taking the fear out of HVS and giving yourself power over it, is to tell five people you know about it. Explain the syndrome, its effects, and how you handle it. Unraveling the tight spiral of HVS can be a long, yet illuminating process. Gaining insight into the mechanisms that bring on HVS symptoms is only the starting point though.

Once you have grasped this point, plenty of help is available out in the community to help you rebuild a healthy self-image, if you need it. Family, individual, and group counseling is available from a variety of agencies. Check out your local library for information, and browse through the dozens of excellent self-help books on the shelves. Coming to grips with HVS, and getting it off your chest, will put you back in the driver's seat and in—not under or out—of control.

Further Reading
"Exhaustion: Cardiac Rehabilitation's Starting Point,"
   P. G. F. Nixon, *Physiotherapy Journal*, May 1986.
Feel the Fear and Do It Anyway, Susan Jeffries (Century,
   London, 1989).

SEVEN
Total Body Relaxation

Hyperventilators who may have been struggling for months, even years, with over-breathing, bizarre symptoms, fear, and tension, find it extremely hard to let go and relax. Releasing physical tension helps let go of mental stress—the rats-in-the-brain repetitive thoughts that go round and round in the mind. This negative internal chatterbox can be just as hard to subdue as trigger-happy lungs.

Learning the knack of switching on relaxation if familiar HVS symptoms reappear is an effective way of stopping the condition in its tracks. It may be difficult at first to feel confident that you can release tension, and to take time for yourself to practice relaxation techniques. But daily relaxation does help unknot your life. It gives you more reserves to cope with daily stresses—good and bad—that are part of normal life.

Choosing a suitable relaxation method

All relaxation techniques start with low, slow diaphragmatic breathing, so mastering Chapter 5 is essential before continuing further with learning total body relaxation.

There are several methods to choose from. Your choice will depend on whether mental or physical tension is more of a problem, and where you are at the time. Knowing different methods makes you more adaptable. Most public hospital physiotherapy outpatient departments teach various types of relaxation as part of general stress management.

To get started, try the *Hyperventilator's Special*, or *Prone Lying Relaxation* (lying on your front).

This method especially suits people who at first feel vulnerable or ill-at-ease trying to learn to relax lying on their backs. Lying face down has a built-in sense of safety, with the soft "under-belly" protected by the "tough shell," or spine.

The main elements of relaxation can be practiced. These include:

- Diaphragmatic breathing.
- Switching off antigravity or posture reflexes.
- Arousing awareness of tension areas in the body.
- Reducing entropy of the body. (Entropy is the measurement of energy or heat generated in the body not used for work. Think of a tense person perched on the edge of a chair, using ten times more energy than necessary to keep upright.)

Learning to recognize stress zones in various groups of muscles helps heighten awareness of the powerful switch conscious relaxation can be.

Preparation
- Set aside a time—at least 15 to 20 minutes.
- Choose a quiet place in which to practice.
- Take the telephone off the hook, or turn down the bell volume.

- Tell people around you what you are going to do and why, and ask them not to disturb you for that time. Even very young children can learn to be cooperative about "your time." Some may even enjoy being time-keeper.
- Schedule regular times for practice instead of "finding" time.

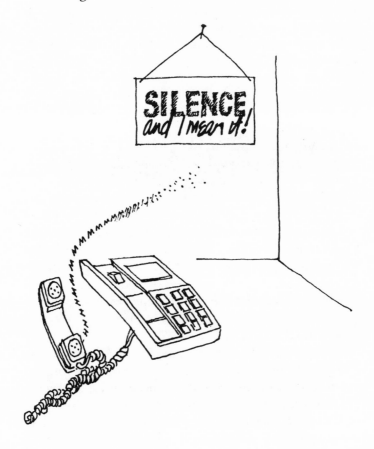

Technique

Lying face down on a firm bed or on the floor, place a rolled blanket or firm pillow under your hips (to free the diaphragm) and under your ankles. You may need a soft pillow under your upper chest if you have a stiff neck.

If you can lie with your arms up, hands under your head, this helps suppress upper-chest breathing (like the forward-leaning rest position). If your shoulders are uncomfortable, keep arms by your sides. *Note:* **Don't go to sleep in this position if you have restricted neck movement.**

PRONE LYING

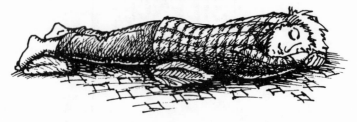

You can practice some of the mental relaxation techniques (below) or listen to soothing music. After an initial concentration on breathing low and slow for three or four breaths, forget about your chest and . . . let go. Relaxing in this position is surprisingly rejuvenating.

Progressive Physical Relaxation

This involves methodically contracting or stretching big groups of muscles for five to six seconds and letting go for fifteen to twenty seconds, concentrating on feeling the difference between tension and release. This is an excellent way of pinpointing tension zones, such as neck, scalp, shoulders, hands, and lower back. The majority of people taken through Progressive Physical Relaxation are extremely surprised at the amount of physical stress they have been holding on to, and are even more surprised at how good it feels to let it go.

Technique
Lying on your back on a bed or the floor, with a pillow under your head and knees, start with two or three low, slow breaths, then forget your breathing while you gently tighten the muscles of your left ankle, pulling your toes up towards you and pressing your left knee into the pillow to tighten your whole leg to the hip. (Your left heel will lift off the bed.) Hold for five seconds—let go slowly, and relax for 15 to 20 seconds. Repeat with the right leg.

Continue with the same timing as you go on to stretch and elongate the fingers and thumb of your left hand. Let go slowly and... relax. Repeat with the right hand.

Push your left elbow gently into the bed. Let go slowly and... relax. Repeat with your right elbow.

Slide your hands down the bed or floor towards your feet, feeling the stretch to the shoulders and neck muscles. Let go slowly and... relax.

Tuck in your chin and gently press your head back into the pillow, being aware of stretching the long muscles up the back of your neck. Let go slowly and... relax.

Very lightly, bring your teeth together. With lips remaining closed, separate your teeth a little and push your lower jaw forward... and relax... being aware of your tongue resting on the floor of your mouth, not clenched up against the roof.

Screw up your nose... and let go and... relax.

Think of your eyelids as light as feathers, resting softly over your eyes. With eyes remaining closed, raise your eyebrows as high as you can... and let go slowly... feeling your brow and scalp smooth and relaxed. There is commonly a lot of tension held here. Repeat two or three times.

Imagine all tension leaving your body through the top of your head.

Check tension zones, and repeat sequences in those areas that still feel tight. You may have to repeat tensing / relaxing routines ten or more times in some stressy areas before you feel release.

When you feel you have unwound physically, rest and enjoy the feeling. Keep nagging or disruptive thoughts out of your mind by focusing on neutral repetitive ones— mentally chanting your two-times tables, for example.

The whole process usually takes 15 to 20 minutes. When it is time to stop (checking your watch will not disturb relaxation), take two or three low, slow breaths and have a good stretch before *slowly* getting up.

Adapting this method to sitting upright in a chair is easy, and can be used at work or on planes, buses, or trains.

To learn the sequences, it may help to ask someone to read out the orders for you, or to tape yourself reading the sequences—with timing—to play back to yourself, perhaps with soothing music to follow. *Music for Airports* by Brian Eno, with its slow, rhythmic, ethereal sounds, is an excellent example of "switching off" music.

Mental relaxation techniques
The most popular methods are:

Passive Mental Relaxation
This involves sitting comfortably, eyes closed, hands on thighs, palms of the hands turned up, and after the first three or four low, slow breaths, not thinking about breathing or trying to relax but passively accepting whatever floats through the mind. Concentration is focused by silent repetition of sounds (for example, repeating the word "one" with each breath out). Along with mental relaxation, a deep physical relaxation is experienced as well.

Transcendental Meditation (TM)
Based on the above technique, an individual word is given, to be repeatedly silently and rapidly, focusing on deep physical and mental relaxation. Nagging conscious thoughts are pushed out by the silent repetition of your word. Most major towns have a TM center. Introduced to the West nearly 30 years ago, it has remained a popular relaxation/meditation method. Although it is relatively expensive, people who have difficulty getting started with relaxation may enjoy the group support.

Auto Hypnosis
This mental relaxation method involves sitting fully supported in a chair about three meters from a wall, and

focusing on a spot slightly above eye-level. Counting breaths back from 100, picture yourself "floating" and "free." As your eyes start to feel heavy, let them close, and stop counting when you feel floppy and pleasantly relaxed.

You will be fully awake and aware of your surroundings and able to check your watch, to time your relaxation. When you want to finish, count three breaths to slowly revert to normal, while holding on to the pleasant relaxed feeling.

Creative Visualization
Setting yourself up as for other methods (sitting, or lying on your back or stomach), creative visualization involves relaxing around positive and pleasurable mental images. By mentally involving all your senses—imagining tastes, smells, textures, and sounds—you build up a rich picture in your mind. Remembering, for example, a childhood picnic with the sounds of the sea, hot sun on your skin (without having to worry about sunscreen!), sand between your toes, the smell and textures of peeling an orange, and the sweet taste of its flesh, can be physically and mentally relaxing.

Taking time to build up a rich, complex, pleasurable picture can also include creative visualizations of positive actions taken by you to release tension, such as imagining slowly and methodically unknotting a rope bound around your problems.

About two-billion brain cells make up our speech and conscious thought centers. But our unconscious is made up of 100-billion brain cells, and our visual sense operates mainly in this larger area. No one has worked out why, but our brains do not differentiate between vividly imagined events and real ones. When you think about a painful or frightening situation, your body reacts as though it was really happening (as in the Think Test). Recent experiments on the muscles of people with back pain show that muscle tension increased between two and six times when the person being tested simply *thought* about their pain. Reversing this response makes sense. Relaxation with visualization is a very potent natural relaxant.

BODY SYSTEMS	DURING RELAXATION	UNDER STRESS
Breathing rate	Down	Up
Heart rate	Down	Up
Blood pressure	Down	Up
Blood supply to muscles and organs	Up	Down
Muscle tension	Down	Up
Adrenalin output	Down	Up, Up, Up

Other methods of relaxation

Joining a yoga class is an excellent way of combining exercise, breathing, and relaxation all in one. Most classes finish with a 20-30-minute total body and mind relaxation session. Some classes teach meditation techniques for home practice as well. Joining a class is often the best way for busy people to schedule, without guilt, time for themselves. Shop around and find a class that suits you.

Treating yourself to a regular back or full-body massage from a reputable masseur is an excellent alternative to the more cerebral approaches to relaxation. People who have been long-time hyperventilators frequently have stiff, tense upper spines and knotty muscles with painful trigger points. Having these gently kneaded and loosened up can make you feel as though you have had three relaxation sessions and a good night's sleep rolled into one.

Having a facial is another way of taking time for yourself to relax.

Dubbed by one wit as "wooden Valium," rocking back and forth in a rocking chair is a tried and true method of relaxing, from infancy through to old age. Many people recovering from HVS swear by this as a "quick-fix" relaxation method.

How often—how long?

Feeling good enough about yourself to make regular relaxation a priority is important, because regular practice is essential. To start with, you may not feel much immediate benefit; it is often other people who remark on changes and improvements.

The ideal is to weave two 15- to 20-minute relaxation sessions into your day. Experiment with different methods for different times of the day and week. Sometimes, in the early days, unpleasant reactions to letting go puts hyperventilators off continuing with relaxation, but it is worth persevering. HVS feeds on tension and anxiety.

Regular practice increases your general awareness of stresses and strains and the need to let go shoulders and upper-chest muscles. Learning to do "mini-relaxes"— checking and releasing tension zones at the same time as you check your breathing pattern with the Lung Ho salute—is of enormous value too.

Just as you recognize triggers that bring on hyperventilation, create come relaxation triggers of your own to combat it. Small things such as mentally repeating the phrase "Lips together, jaw relaxed, breathing low and slow," turning your palms up and letting your shoulders relax, or pressing stress-releasing trigger points in the muscles on the backs of your hands between the thumb and index finger help switch off tension.

Remind yourself how much energy you are wasting by being physically tense, and that physical tension goes hand-in-hand with the negative mental chatterbox that constantly undermines your feelings of well-being.

Remind yourself that *relaxation only helps eliminate the symptoms not the causes of stress.* Develop the ability to "accept the things you cannot change, have the courage to change the things you can, and the wisdom to know the difference" (to borrow from the Alcoholics Anonymous prayer). Addiction to bad breathing can be a hard habit to break.

Check your shoulders, elbows, and hands when walking, and make sure they are not clenched and tight. If they are, it means you are carrying your stress with you, like heavy unwanted baggage.

Look in your local library for books and tapes on relaxation.

Make regular total-body relaxation as important as cleaning your teeth.

Further Reading
The Relaxation Response, Herbert Benson (Fount Paperbacks, London, 1977).

Simple Relaxation, Laura Mitchell (John Murray, London, 1988).

Super Health, booklet and tape, available from Mental Health Foundation branches.

Visualisation for Change, Patrick Fanning (New Harbinger Press, Oakland, 1988).

EIGHT
Talk

Talking can be a major problem for over-breathers for two reasons. The first is breath control while speaking (and the one thing you really need to be able to do, through the power of speech, is to express ideas and emotions—to your doctor and to people close to you). Using quick, gasping upper-chest mouth breaths while talking can trigger HVS symptoms. Slightly husky, light speech, punctuated by throat-clearing, sniffing, sighing, or yawning often indicates hyperventilation. Marilyn Monroe's sexy, breathless voice may have had more to do with an overactive upper chest—her waist pinioned by a cinch belt—than with true desire! A full-toned confident voice needs good breath control: ask any politician, actor, or singer.

Tips for breath control while speaking:

- Relax your shoulders and low, slow nose-breathe before speaking.
- Draw air in through your nose between sentences while talking, instead of quickly gulping in air through your mouth.
- Mentally put commas and pauses into your speech.
- Practice speaking in front of a mirror. Recite the alphabet or two-times tables. Use the Lung Ho salute to check chest movement.

- Remember to swallow or breath-hold for two to three seconds if you get an irresistible urge to yawn, sigh, or take a big breath.
- Watch other people's breathing patterns when they speak. Listen during telephone conversations. See if you can spot another hyperventilator. Game shows and television soap operas take on a whole new meaning when you look for good and bad breathers.
- Always be aware of centering your breathing—low and slow.

Combining eating and talking with breath control is a big problem for some people. Most of the best advice about relaxed eating was taught to us as infants by our parents:

- Always sit down to eat. *Never eat on the run.*
- Avoid talking with your mouth full.
- Nose-breathe while chewing.
- Eat slowly.
- Eat very small mouthfuls.
- Chew thoroughly.
- Never eat slumped in a low chair.
- Drink slowly, too, holding your breath as you sip, to prevent air-gulping.

If breath control while speaking or eating continues to be a problem, seek expert advice from a speech therapist.

The second area where talking may be difficult is when trying to voice deep anxieties about HVS symptoms. Bottling up problems is not good for your health. Anxiety increases mental and physical tension and adrenalin output, revving up the heart and breathing rates, and HVS. Recent research has scientifically proved that thinking or talking about physical symptoms can both directly and indirectly affect the body's physiology—a fact known unscientifically since the dawn of time. (An example of the direct effect of thought on physiology is, of course, the Think Test.) The indirect physiological effect lies in the relationship between stress and depression. Experiencing loss of control over parts of your life (as felt with HVS) is a major ingredient in depression. A sense of isolation develops if you are afraid of confiding in anyone (worse still if you do, and are disbelieved or thought neurotic). Lacking confidence to cope socially or keep up friendships, or thinking you are letting family, friends, or workmates down is a common sign of anxiety and a potent depressant.

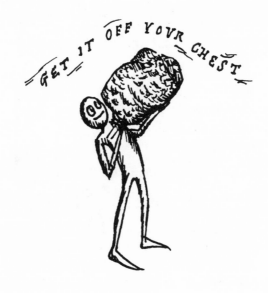

Listening skills often need brushing up too. Expression and communication are very much two-way processes. People close to you may have become alarmed, confused, or even bored by your real and imagined disorders. Relaxing enough to be able to listen to other people is as necessary as finding someone who will listen to you.

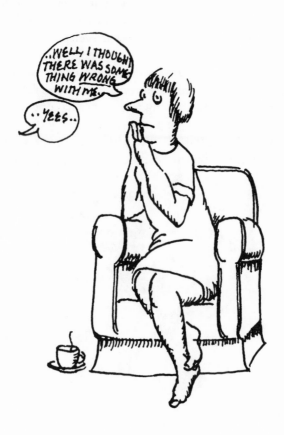

Scientific medicine, with hi-tech surgical and pharmaceutical interventions, has revolutionized the "healing arts" over the last 20 years. But it has also produced a society that holds an unrealistic belief in drugs as the cure-all, instilling a passive attitude to becoming well. Recovery from HVS requires an active involvement and personal commitment. And talking—being able to identify problems and confront the need for acceptance or change—is a vital part of reducing stress and being in, not under, control.

For those who have difficulty identifying the sources of anxiety, sessions with a clinical psychologist, psychiatrist, or therapist may be of enormous benefit in speeding up recovery.

Regaining a resonant confident voice comes with low, slow breathing, relaxation and talking out, and releasing bottled-up resentments and emotions.

Find someone you trust to confide in. Use positive language, and, starting with the next breath, talk yourself up and away from HVS.

Further Reading

Listen to Me, Listen to You, Anne Kotzman (Penguin Books, Melbourne, 1989).

Mental Health for Women, Hilary Haines (Reed Methuen, Auckland, 1985).

Will the Real Mr. New Zealand Please Stand Up?, Gwendoline Smith (Penguin Books, Auckland, 1990).

NINE
Exercise

Hyperventilation Syndrome and low physical fitness tend to go hand-in-hand. The effects of inactivity—sluggish circulation, flabby muscles, lack of energy, and shortness of breath—all add to a general loss of self-confidence.

This is most often due to:

- Fear of triggering uncontrollable rapid breathing during effort.
- Panic about not being able to draw the next breath in.
- The side effects of poor sleep and depression.
- Fear of fatigue.

Nearly all chronic hyperventilators complain of muscle fatigue. The most common types complained of are central fatigue, with generalized feelings of low energy; and peripheral fatigue, felt in the limbs, where muscles tire easily and protest.

Why is physical fitness important in HVS?

Physical fitness is described in the "Teachers' Guide for Fitness for Living" *(Clinical Management,* vol. 9, no. 3) as "the body's ability to meet the normal demands of everyday life—work and recreation—with ease, and with enough margin to adequately cope with emergencies." Most hyperventilators would admit falling far behind this description.

Everybody feels better when they have reserves of energy to spare. Feeling fit has added bonuses. It leads to improvement of body image and a stronger sense of self-reliance. Enjoyment of regular physical exercise and the sense of confidence it brings is a vital part of banishing HVS.

Does it have to be vigorous?

The three main ingredients in a recipe to improve physical fitness are:

- Endurance exercise. This trains the body to work for long periods of time, by improving heart and circulation (cardiovascular) fitness (e.g., running, jogging, or aerobics classes).
- Strengthening exercise. Specific groups of muscles are trained to improve function and prevent injury during particular leisure- or work-related effort (e.g., leg-muscle strengthening for skiers).
- Flexibility exercise. Joints and muscles are kept supple and able to move through a full range of movement, to prevent muscle imbalances that might lead to injury or, in the long term, osteo-arthritis (e.g., dance, stretch, or yoga classes, and swimming).

While all three ingredients are important in a balanced fitness program, emphasis in recent times has leaned towards the cardiovascular. The fitness boom of the last decade has given the impression that to become fit means being encased in spandex and working out in gyms. Many people torture their bodies into fitness levels way beyond their needs, but the byproduct of this—feeling healthy and on top of the world—keeps them at it.

The risk of injury in these endurance-based, high-impact pastimes is high, especially if previously unfit people take them on without preparation. During high-impact exercise, such as aerobics and running, the feet hit the ground with a force between two and four times the body weight. You need to be *basically* fit even to start these, in order to avoid strains, sprains, and pain.

Low-impact exercise—brisk walking, cycling, low-resistance circuit training (if you want to join a gym), and swimming—is a great way to improve fitness for the average person's needs. There are plenty of other options: gardening, playing outdoor games with your kids, going dancing, or walking the dog are all excellent "body boosters."

Getting started

Hyperventilators tend to be overachievers. Make sure progress is gradual. Take it easy. Include a friend or partner who knows about your symptoms to "fitten up" with you.

Start with walking, which is a safe, enjoyable, and easy way to achieve *basic* fitness. It's cheap, interesting (looking at your surroundings), needs no special clothes except for a comfortable pair of walking shoes, and a big advantage is that you can nose-breathe while doing it.

(If you have an aversion to outdoor exercise, hiring or buying an exercycle is a good alternative. Increase cycling times as you would with walking.)

Set yourself a time, not distance, to walk (or exercycle). Decide for yourself, based on your symptoms, and err

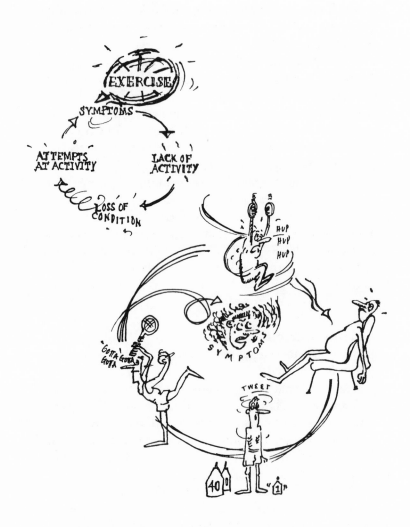

on the light side at first. (Some start as low as three minutes—one-and-a-half-minutes out, one-and-a-half back—if walking.)

If you start with walking or cycling times of less than ten minutes, do two sessions—one in the morning and one in the afternoon—until you can do ten minutes easily at each session.

At first, limit yourself to walking on the flat. Include hills as you start to feel fitter and more confident. Take smaller strides and *slow down*.

Check that your shoulders and arms are relaxed and loose. Use a good arm swing and walk at a brisk pace.

If you start to want to mouth-breathe, feel breathless, or experience chest symptoms, stop immediately and take up a rest position—sit on a fence or wall, or stand with your arms on a car roof, partner's shoulders, or a fence, and low, slow nose-breathe your way back to normal. Use the Lung Ho salute to check breathing pattern and rate.

Undoubtedly, some days will be harder than others and you must be prepared for ups and downs. Gradually your tolerance to exercise and your ability to control breathing will improve.

When you reach a level where you can walk briskly for twenty minutes every day with few or no breathless problems, you will have reached a basic level of fitness.

If you are quite happy to keep on with brisk walking, three or four 30- to 40-minute walks a week are enough to *maintain* basic fitness.

The joys of walking include:

- Aerobic benefits (heart/lung efficiency) are achieved after only fifteen minutes of brisk walking.

- Digestion and bowel function are toned up.
- Sleeping patterns improve.
- It is very relaxing.

For variety, include other ways of keeping fit:

- Use the stairs at work. At first, walk up one or down two flights before getting the lift. Increase by one flight a week (to a maximum five up, ten down).
- Try a rebounder, bouncing to your favorite music.
- Yoga and t'ai chi classes are especially recommended, combining breathing, exercise (especially flexibility), and relaxation.
- Whacking games—tennis, badminton, and squash—are good for people who need to release anger or resentments.
- Swimming—some may need coaching to help with breathing.

Eating and exercise

If you are overweight, regular exercise helps weight loss. Many people mistakenly think that exercise makes you eat more. In fact, you feel less like eating directly after exercise, so if you are trying to lose weight, exercising shortly before meals helps tone down the appetite.

If you are very underweight, take care to avoid heavy-endurance types of exercise, and concentrate on flexibility and low-resistance activities two to three hours before meals.

Good nutrition is an important part of fitness. Many authorities cite poor nutrition as a major source of stress. If you have been feeling depressed, not eating properly or not getting enough exercise, physical neglect feeds your depression. This drastically increases the potential for sickness and misery.

Skipping meals and relying on "comfort" foods like chocolate bars to boost flagging energy levels will only add to an already overburdened nervous system. Hyperventilators tend to interpret their fatigue symptoms as being due to low blood sugar (hypoglycemia—a fashionable complaint). But sugar is not, and never has been, an essential part of our diet. The sugar "high" after eating sweets is short-lived. The body's production of the hormone insulin soon clears the high blood-sugar level and works to restore a normal balance, resulting in a further slump in energy. Reaching for more sugar only repeats the cycle. Choose protein snacks instead—a few nuts or a small slice of cheese, for instance.

High sugar intake, whether from sweet foods or too much alcohol, tends to accelerate your heartrate, fueling HVS. While one glass of wine is an excellent relaxant, more may be asking for trouble.

Smoking

Smoking is another habit that complicates a hyperventilator's life. It is not hard to imagine the chaos that strong inhalations of smoke wreak upon your already "hyper" breathing.

Try to give up smoking while you are retraining your breathing patterns. Join a smoke cessation group. See if you can spot fellow hyperventilators. Ridding the body of nicotine takes only about forty-eight hours, which for most people is a manageable time to go through the hell of breaking the nicotine habit by the "cold turkey" technique. Nicotine patches or short, decreasing courses of nicotine chewing gum can help control nasty withdrawal symptoms.

It is usually more difficult to give up the *rituals* of smoking, and for hyperventilators that includes the over-breath of an inhalation. Every time you think of the pleasures of smoking, give equal time to acknowledging the harmful effects and what it is doing to your heart and breathing rates. Consider whether smoking is an excuse to hyperventilate.

Think about what kind of smoker you are:

- If you smoke to relax, try total body relaxation instead.
- If you smoke to give yourself a lift, get out in the fresh air or do some exercise instead.
- If you smoke because of the ritual of handling cigarettes or other smoking paraphernalia, invest in some worry beads to occupy your hands.

Remember: smoking heavily is asking for trouble.
Stopping is best.
Cutting down helps.

Regular exercise helps release naturally occurring opiopeptides into the bloodstream that make you feel good. Bones are kept strong too, especially important for post-menopausal women, or those on courses of steroids.

Regular enjoyable exercise builds reserves against HVS. Keeping fit helps conquer panicky feelings. Movement and pleasure in physical action is a very basic human need. Enjoyable exercise is very much a part of recovery.

Further Reading

Body Sense, Vernon Coleman (Thames and Hudson, London, 1984).

"Hyperventilation Syndrome and Muscle Fatigue," H. Folgering and A. Snik, *Journal of Psychosomatic Research,* vol. 32, no. 2, 1988.

"The Natural Exercise Prescription," Z. Altug and M. Miller, *Clinical Management,* vol. 9, no. 3.

TEN
Rest and Sleep

Adequate rest and sleep are vital to good health. One of the most common HVS symptoms people complain of is erratic sleep and vivid or bad dreams. Sound sleep provides a total release from the pressures of daily life, so to be deprived of satisfying sleep can cause a great deal of distress and anxiety to an already stretched nervous system.

Very few people get through life without experiencing muddled sleep patterns, either from extremes of happiness or despair. Someone newly in love hardly seems to need any sleep at all, and feels no worse for it. But during periods of ill-health the body demands more sleep. Anxiety and fear about the symptoms of HVS may be one reason for sleeplessness. But the vivid dreams and nightmares, where the hyperventilator wakes with a pounding heart and a sense of panic, can make sleep itself fearful.

Normal sleep
Sleep is controlled from a regulating center deep in the brain stem. It processes messages from all over the body—joints, muscles, organs—as well as from the higher thought centers in the brain—to either induce sleep (low levels of stimulation to the sleep regulating center) or wakefulness (high levels of stimulation). So a calm mind as well as a relaxed body is needed for satisfying sleep.

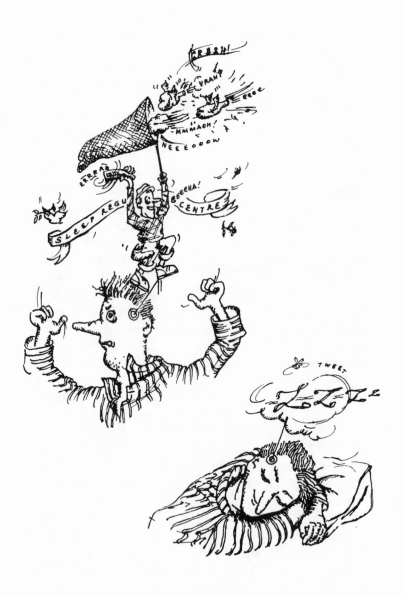

Sleep goes through cycles of quiet sleep, which is true rest with a *quiet* brain. This cycle lasts about an hour. This is followed by rapid eye movement (REM) sleep, a shorter cycle of about 20 to 30 minutes where the brain is very *active*. This is dream time.

During quiet sleep, the body's metabolic rate, blood pressure, and heart rate become slightly lowered, and the breathing rate is deep and regular. In REM sleep, the heart beats up to five percent faster, there is a slight increase in blood pressure and metabolic rate, the eyes dart about under closed lids, and breathing becomes irregular. The average sleep needed for an adult is seven and a half hours—five complete quiet plus REM sleep cycles. Individual needs vary widely of course according to age, health, and personality.

Why do people with HVS have sleep problems?
For people with HVS, who are sensitive to even very small drops in carbon dioxide levels in their blood, the irregular breathing during REM sleep acts on the unconscious mind, producing vivid or nightmarish dreams and lack of satisfying sleep. Stress levels, high enough during waking hours, are added to by disturbed rest and anxiety over poor sleep. The downward spiral started by wakefulness, worry, nightmares, and sleeplessness can take a long time, and a lot of patience and understanding, to spiral up and away from.

The Good Sleep Plan
If you are dependent on sleeping pills, the following will be of little use. While sleeping pills can be a blessing for a

short time, if used continuously for more than two weeks they cease to work. They are addictive; withdrawal from them should be gradual and undertaken with skilled help. Only use the Good Sleep Plan once you have decided to make a success of getting off the "little blue pills."

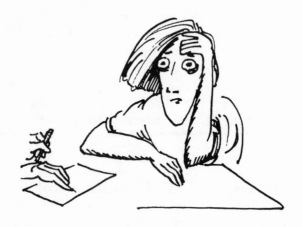

Try these simple strategies, and give yourself time to re-establish a good sleep routine. Let your family and friends know your plans. If you share your bed, your partner will definitely need to know!

- Make your bedroom a stress-free zone. No television, telephone, or noisy clocks.
- Small changes, such as new bed linen or moving the bed, can help start the new routine and break old associations.
- Soft, low lighting helps create a restful atmosphere.
- Use the bed for sleeping only.

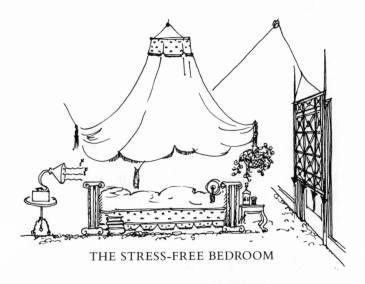

THE STRESS-FREE BEDROOM

- No reading, eating, sewing, writing letters, talking on the phone.
- Making love is an exception. Good sex is a powerful prelude to relaxed sleep. Unfortunately, deep post-orgasmic relaxation lasts only four or five minutes, so if you haven't fallen asleep by then it is of no added benefit. Seek expert help if anxiety about sex is a problem.
- Avoid rich, heavy, or late-night dinners, or Chinese food (high in monosodium glutamate) at the end of the day.
- Cut out coffee and strong tea for a month. Try decaffeinated. Reintroduce it gradually after a month, and even then, try and avoid it after 4 p.m. If you are a heavy coffee drinker, be prepared for withdrawal symptoms such as irritability and shakiness. Drink plenty of water.

- Avoid television news and talkback radio for a month. Watch only light or funny programs or videos. Reduce extremes of negative and positive stimulation in the three or four hours before sleep.
- Exercise. As noted in Chapter 9, exercise helps induce sleep. It should be within four or five hours of bedtime.
- Have a warm bath before going to bed.
- Fix a regular time to go to bed and to get up in the morning. *Never go to bed earlier or get up later than those appointed times.*
- Never have day sleeps. Daytime tiredness is more often caused by boredom or lack of activity. Go for a stroll instead of snoozing.
- Try warm milk as a nightcap. Milk has high levels of tryptophan,★ a naturally occurring enzyme that the body digests and converts into serotonin. This "sleep nectar" has a powerful influence in promoting good moods and sound sleep.
- Sedative herb teas such as pasaflora or chamomile are safe alternatives for those who cannot tolerate milk.
- Write a list of things to be remembered or done the next day, so you don't worry about tomorrow, today. Constant projecting into the future is a sure-fire sleep-killer.
- Never go to bed on an unresolved fight or argument.

★ Tryptophan has been available in tablet form, and has been used for over 25 years in New Zealand as a non-addictive, natural alternative to sleeping pills. Recent research in the U.S. and Europe has shown that high dosages may be linked to a sometimes fatal blood disorder; contaminated stocks are thought to be a possible cause of the problem. While there is doubt, rely on dietary intake of tryptophan (protein foods like milk, poultry, meat, fish, and cheese are rich sources).

Getting off to sleep

Based on the sleep-retraining method devised by Dr. Richard Bootzin of the U.S., the following regime is extremely successful. People who have tried this scheme and stuck to it find it takes between two and six weeks to start working, and feel it is well worth the effort in restoring refreshing drug-free sleep.

- Once prepared and into bed, practice low, slow diaphragmatic breathing (through the nose) and relaxation techniques. Check for tension areas and let them go.
- In a comfortable sleeping position (side-lying), glance at the time and if after 15 minutes you are still awake, get out of bed. Go into another room and do something else (read, watch a funny video, play Patience, listen to soothing music). When you feel ready to sleep, go back to bed, and if again you are not asleep within 15 minutes, repeat the sequence until you do. Try this approach to early-morning waking as well. *Learn to associate bed with sleep—if you're not sleeping, don't stay in bed.*

If your appointed waking time happens to come in the middle of a deep, quiet sleep cycle, you may find it hard to wake up. Don't interpret that as "waking up tired." If your appointed waking time comes towards the end of REM sleep cycle, you will wake up more alert and with fleeting memories of dreams. But if nightmares wake you with hyperventilation symptoms, get up and recover in the sitting rest position (see page 41), concentrating hard on relaxing your neck and shoulders, and nose-breathing low and slow. Soothing music helps too. When your breathing is under control and your heart rate has slowed down, try going back to sleep, knowing hyperventilation is the problem and you have the power to control it.

A large part of success in restoring good sleep patterns is change of attitude. People who go to bed expecting *not* to sleep, are usually proved right. Breathing control and relaxation will remove hyperventilation-induced symptoms.

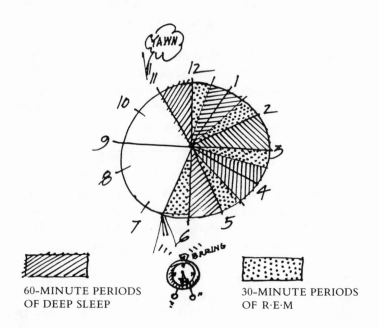

60-MINUTE PERIODS
OF DEEP SLEEP

30-MINUTE PERIODS
OF R·E·M

The bad sleep pattern can be broken, and a new refreshing one restored.

A few people never manage to establish normal sleep patterns. If you are one of these, at least make it anxiety-free time and use the extra hours of wakefulness creatively and with acceptance.

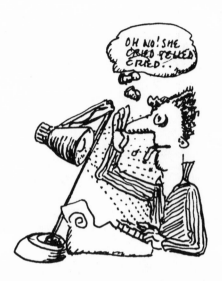

Further Reading

Getting to Sleep, Ellen Mohr Catalauo (New Harbinger Publications, Oakland, 1990).

A Good Night's Sleep, J. S. Maxem (W. W. Norton, New York and London, 1981).

Natural Sleep (How to Get Your Share), P. Goldberg and D. Kaufman (Rodale Press, Emmaus, Pennsylvania, 1978).

ELEVEN
What can Family and Friends do to Help a Hyperventilator?

Learn to be a very good listener.

Always use positive language—"Let your shoulders go" rather than "Don't tense your shoulders," or "Breathe low and slow" instead of "Don't breathe so fast." If you meet irritation at your observations, apologize and back off.

Discuss "flash points" at home or at work where tensions are highest, and see if they can be avoided, confronted, or shared.

Use touch instead of words where possible. A gentle massage of tense shoulders can be far better than words. Scalp massages sooth tension headaches and tight scalp muscles. Hand and foot massages are also good diversions.

Try not to be over-protective. This can be very difficult, especially with children and teenagers. If someone close to you does have a bad spell, let them get on with their new coping strategies.

Encourage rest / relaxation times. Hyperventilators often feel guilty about needing time to relax. Help them recognize that not only are they helping themselves, but their family / partner / friends as well.

If you live with someone whose self-esteem is very low and they have become socially isolated, a gradual reentry into the outside world is best initiated by the hyperventilator themselves, as they start to feel more in control. Realize it may take a long time. Don't push or nag.

Try to keep stimulation levels down at stressful times. For example, invest in headphones if someone in the household insists on listening to the Stranglers at full volume while someone else is trying to relax. Be thoughtful about noise and social pressures. Avoid stressful topics at mealtimes.

Above all, relax.

Ideal gifts for a hyperventilator
A sheepskin underlay for the bed.
Worry beads.
Walking shoes.
A funny video.
A copy of the *Bumper Book of Jokes*.
A course of massages.
A recording of Roger Eno's *Voices*.

TWELVE
The Last Word

A final, and encouraging story from M, a 39-year-old woman with HVS:

Even though on the outside I always looked a fairly laid-back sort of person, I've absorbed an awful lot of stress in my time. About eight or nine years ago I started to be not so . . . resilient.

On the surface I had it all: good marriage, husband a success object, two great kids, and an interesting part-time job. Total fulfillment, you'd think. But after a slight accident, when I fell down some steps and had a period of back pain and sleeping badly, I started getting uptight and panicky about minor things. The kids were little then, and I found that pretty stressful. Besides feeling vaguely unwell, I was aware of my breathing—feeling that all the air was pushing up in my chest, trying to stop me breathing. I talked about these symptoms to my doctor. He didn't say much, but when he was out of the room I peeped at his notes and saw that he'd written "Anxiety attacks" to describe my symptoms. I felt terrible—it reinforced my lack of self-confidence, which was already at an all-time low.

The crunch came a few months later when one day at home, out of the blue, I felt hot and clammy, heart racing and breathless, for no reason. I crawled to bed but felt I couldn't get flat enough; I wanted to press myself on the floor. I managed to telephone my husband and whisper, "I'm dying"—I really thought I was. The feelings of flying apart, absolute terror, falling down through the world, spinning through the universe... was the worst thing I'd ever experienced.

My GP gave me a course of sleeping pills and Serapax tranquilizers to take if I had any more "attacks." Even though the Serapax took 20 minutes to work, I knew I'd be okay and I relaxed.

For the last four years I haven't been able to go out without a bottle of Serapax in my bag. Over the last year, since starting treatment, I've hardly had to use them. And last week I achieved a major breakthrough: I felt confident enough in my ability to control my breathing to leave the pills at home.

After years of clinging on, being "clenched" all the time, when you do let go a lot of things happen. After the initial glow of having HVS diagnosed—that there is something wrong and it *can* be fixed—I had a time of feeling worse. I found it really hard learning to relax, to take time for myself and make it a priority. The whole family has had to adapt to these changes.

It's taken about eight months for me to feel that I've recovered. I sleep pretty well now, and I don't panic if I have a bad night. I use visualizations a lot. Before going to sleep I relax by imagining a big soda bottle in my chest, and I slowly unscrew the top, letting out the built-up pressure little by little until it's all gone. By then my breathing is low and slow and I feel good. When I relax lying on my stomach I visualize a nasty little gnome squeezing my upper-back muscles with knobbly hands. I concentrate on those hands and watch them loosen their grip, let go, stop controlling me, and disappear. Imagining slowly unraveling a tightly knotted rope is useful when I'm out and about.

I feel really glad not to be dependent on pills any more. I feel better being fitter and having physical reserves again.

Whenever the going gets tough I just think about... my next breath!

Conclusion

Hyperventilation Syndrome is alive and thriving in the 1990s. Diagnosis and definition have been contentious issues in recent years and are still the subject of lively debate amongst doctors. However, many sufferers have responded to treatments involving breathing retraining and relaxation, and have enjoyed the far-reaching benefits of balanced blood gases and pH levels.

Six weeks of following the BETTER breathing plan should start to give good results. Fifty percent of the cure is knowing about and understanding the nature of HVS. The rest is up to you. Remember, it will take time.

To start out, work on breathing—pattern first then rate and relaxation. Tune into your breathing regularly, concentrating on "Lips together, jaw relaxed, breathing low and slow."

If relaxation seems pointless at first, keep practicing. You will soon appreciate its importance.

Organize family and friends so that you can start the sleep regime as soon as possible.

Start exercising only when your breathing is consistently low and slow, and once you have developed a good relaxation response.

Don't make the mistake of trying to achieve fitness too quickly, even if you have been fit in the past. The aim of movement and activity is *enjoyment*. Watch out for those aggressive and competitive instincts. Put them on hold.

Breathing retraining may take a long time to become a habit. Don't be too hard on yourself if you do go off the rails and lapse into bad breathing. Take a break and use a rest position.

Focus all your attention on . . . the next breath.

Index

NOTES:

NOTES:

NOTES:

NOTES:

NOTES:

NOTES:

WELLNESS... SMALL CHANGES THAT YOU CAN USE
TO MAKE A BIG DIFFERENCE
by John Travis, M.D. and Regina Ryan

Geared to busy people, or those who are not ready to radically change their lifestyle, this book outlines fifty small changes anyone can make in areas including nutrition, relaxation, work, and relationships. The suggestions can be taken together to form a coherent wellness program, or done one at a time as convenient.

$5.95 paper, *80 pages*

WELLNESS WORKBOOK
by John Travis, M.D. and Regina Ryan

An updated edition of one of the first books on total wellness—how to integrate physical, emotional, intellectual, and spiritual factors to create vibrant, life-long health.

$11.95 paper, *256 pages*

HIGH LEVEL WELLNESS
by Donald Ardell

An in-depth examination of the wellness movement, and how it has provided a vital, workable alternative to doctors, drugs, and disease. Describes a wide range of approaches and resources.

$9.95 paper, *384 pages*

HEALING ENVIRONMENTS
by Carol Venolia

This holistic approach to "indoor well-being" examines healing, awareness, and empowerment, and how they are affected by various aspects of our environment. Its principles can be applied to homes, workplaces, and healthcare centers to bring greater peace and harmony into our lives.

$9.95 paper, *224 pages*

YOUR HOME, YOUR HEALTH, AND WELL-BEING
by David Rousseau, W.J. Rea, M.D. and Jean Enwright

"A well-illustrated, thoroughly researched look at home pollutants and how to transform your living space into a more healthful one."
—*East West magazine*

A guide to the many substances in modern homes which can cause irritation, stress, allergies, even severe environmental illness—and what you can do about them.

$14.95 paper, *320 pages*

CHOOSE TO BE HEALTHY
by Susan Smith Jones, Ph.D.

The choices we make in life can greatly increase our health and happiness—this book details how to analyze one's choices about food, exercise, thought, work, and play, and then use this information to create a better, healthier life.

$9.95 paper, *252 pages*

CHOOSE TO LIVE PEACEFULLY
by Susan Smith Jones, Ph.D.

By nurturing our inner selves and living in personal peace, we can help to bring about global change. In this book, Susan Smith Jones explores the many components of a peaceful, satisfying life—including exercise, nutrition, solitude, meditation, ritual, and environmental awareness—and shows how they can be linked to world peace.

$11.95 paper, *320 pages*

RECOVERY FROM ADDICTION
by John Finnegan and Daphne Grey

Alternative herbal and nutritional therapies for a wide range of addictions, from cigarettes to sugar to caffeine to hard drugs. Includes first-person accounts of how these treatments have worked for a variety of specific problems.

$9.95 paper, *192 pages*

THE PMS SELF-HELP BOOK
by Susan Lark, M.D.

A wonderful hands-on workbook that helps women identify the causes of common PMS symptoms (anxiety, pain, weight gain, chocolate craving, etc.) and diminish or eliminate them through diet, exercise, acupressure, and other drug-free methods.

$14.95 paper, *240 pages*

THE MENOPAUSE SELF-HELP BOOK
by Susan Lark, M.D.

A woman's guide to feeling wonderful for the second half of her life. Explains how and why a woman's body and moods change with menopause, and offers a practical, natural master plan for preventing or relieving negative symptoms.

$14.95 paper, *240 pages*

LOVE IS LETTING GO OF FEAR
by Gerald Jampolsky, M.D.

The lessons in this extremely popular little book (over 1,000,000 in print), based on *A Course in Miracles*, will teach you to let go of fear and remember that our true essence is love. Includes daily exercises.

$7.95 paper or $9.95 cloth, *144 pages*

GENTLE YOGA
by Lorna Bell, R.N. and Eudora Seyfer

This book is especially designed for people with arthritis, stroke damage, or multiple sclerosis, those in wheelchairs, or anyone who needs a gentle, practical way to improve their health through exercise. The book is spiralbound to stay open while you work and includes over 135 helpful illustrations.

$7.95 spiral, *144 pages*

EMBRACE TIGER, RETURN TO MOUNTAIN
by Chungliang Al Huang

The essence of the art of Tai Chi, presented by one of the world's foremost authorities. Huang's unique perspective is based in a deep yet playful understanding of Eastern tradition coupled with years of training in dance and martial arts.

$12.95 paper, *256 pages*

SELF ESTEEM
by Virginia Satir

A simple and succinct declaration of self worth which serves as inspiration and affirmation for anyone who needs a "quick hit" of positive feelings.

$5.95 paper, *64 pages*

THE COMMON BOOK OF CONSCIOUSNESS
Revised Edition by Diana Saltoon

A beloved sourcebook, newly revised and updated for the 1990s. This guide to leading a whole and centered life shows how to use meditation, exercise, and nutrition to gain a higher consciousness and a full, balanced daily life.

$11.95 paper, *160 pages*

THE MAGICAL CHILD WITHIN YOU
by Bruce Davis, Ph.D.

Building upon Gestalt Therapy, Transactional Analysis, and Primal Therapy, Dr. Davis provides a disarmingly simple and delightfully written look at self-awareness and love. This book shows how to find and nurture the magical child who lives within each of us.

$7.95 paper, *128 pages*

Available from your local bookstore, or order direct from the publisher. Please include $1.25 shipping & handling for the first book, and 50 cents for each additional book. California residents include local sales tax. Write for our free complete catalog of over 400 books and tapes.

Ship to:

Name_____

Address_____

City_____State_____Zip_____

Phone: (   )_____

Celestial Arts
Box 7327
Berkeley, CA 94707
For VISA or Mastercard orders call (510) 845-8414

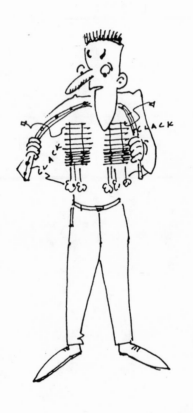

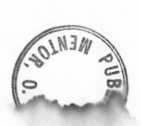